Keto For Vegetarians

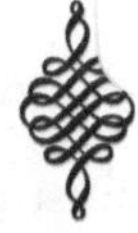

How To Create Ultimate Keto-Vegetarian Lifestyle And Start Losing Weight From Day 1

By

Jamie Knight

purposes only. All effort has been executed to present accurate, up to date, and reliable, complete information. No warranties of any kind are declared or implied. Readers acknowledge that the author is not engaging in the rendering of legal, financial, medical or professional advice. The content within this book has been derived from various sources. Please consult a licensed professional before attempting any techniques outlined in this book.

By reading this document, the reader agrees that under no circumstances are is the author responsible for any losses, direct or indirect, which are incurred as a result of the use of information contained within this document, including, but not limited to, —errors, omissions, or inaccuracies.

Table of Contents

Introduction..1
Chapter One: Ketogenic Diet...7
  Ketosis and Ketogenic Diet......................................9
  How Does A Ketogenic Diet Work?........................11
  Benefits of A Ketogenic Diet.................................13
  Breakdown of Macronutrients.............................15
  Types of Ketogenic Diets.....................................16
  How Will You Know If You Are In Ketosis?..........18
    Testing Ketone Levels In Urine......................19
    Testing Ketone Levels In Breath....................20
    Testing Ketone Levels In The Blood...............20
  How Do You Start A Ketogenic Diet?...................21
Chapter Two: Vegetarian Ketogenic Diet........................24
  Different Types of Vegetarians.............................26
  Vegetarians and Carbs...29
  Keto–Friendly Vegetarian Fats............................35
  Keto–friendly Sources of Vegetarian Protein.......40
    Tofu...40
    Tempeh...41
    Seitan...43
    Seeds and Nuts...43
  The Other Alternatives.......................................45
Chapter Three: How To Get Started?..............................47
  Action Plan...47
    Carb-restriction..48
    Including high-quality protein....................48
    Eat vegetables (at least one to three servings) twice a day.51
    Use plant-based healthy fat oils for salad dressings and cooking.......52
    Seasoning the food with different spices and herbs...........53
  Must-haves (Vegetables, Condiments, Fruit and Spices)........54
    Condiments...56
    Fruit...57
    Spices...57

Meal Ideas for a Vegetarian Ketogenic Diet 59

Chapter Four: Tips and Guidelines **61**

The Do's and Don'ts of KETO 62

Do's of KETO 63

Don'ts of KETO 64

Ways To Avoid Nutrient Deficiencies On A Keto-Vegetarian Diet 65

Vegetarian Keto Shopping List 69

Non-Starchy Vegetables 69

Fruit with low-sugar content 70

Healthy Fats 71

Vegetarian Protein 71

Precautionary Measures To Be Taken On Keto-Veg Diet 72

Chapter Five: Vegetarian Keto Breakfast Recipes **74**

Keto Zucchini Bread with Walnuts 74

Low-carb Cauliflower Hash Browns 76

Keto Coconut Porridge 78

Keto Mushroom Omelet 80

Chapter Six: Vegetarian Keto Lunch Recipes **82**

Crustless Spinach Cheese Pie 82

Rainbow Cauliflower Crust Pizza 84

Roasted Brussels Sprouts with Pecans and Gorgonzola 87

Charred Veggie and Fried Cheese Salad 89

Chapter Seven: Vegetarian Keto Dinner Recipes **91**

5-Minute Keto Pizza 91

Cheese Cauliflower Casserole 93

Vegetarian Lettuce Wraps 94

Mediterranean Roasted Cabbage Steaks with Basil Pesto & Feta 97

Chapter Eight: Vegetarian Keto Snack Recipes **100**

Crunchy Kale Chips 100

Gluten-Free Crispy Buffalo Cauliflower Wings 102

Zucchini Nacho Chips 104

Cabbage Chips 106

Crispy Green Bean Chips 108

Conclusion **110**

Introduction

I would like to take this opportunity to thank you for purchasing this book, "Keto for veg - How To Create The Ultimate Keto-Vegetarian Lifestyle And Start Losing Weight From Day 1."

Are you curious about the Vegetarian Keto diet? Do you want to follow a Keto-Vegetarian lifestyle to manage your weight problems? It is now possible!

It cannot be denied that the vegetarian diet is one of the healthiest diets as it ensures the complete wellness of an individual. Multiples studies have already shown that a proper and well-balanced vegetarian diet can reduce the odds of prevailing diseases such as diabetes, heart disorders, etc. It is believed to improve the health condition in a much more efficient way when compared to a non-vegetarian diet.

However, it cannot be concluded that a vegetarian diet is the best option for everyone's health. For instance, when it comes to weight loss, vegetarians are equally obese just like non-vegetarians. The Ketogenic diet, which is not a vegetarian diet, is more effective when it comes to weight loss. It improves the blood sugar levels and the triglycerides. The Keto diet comes with various health benefits as it was initially discovered to control epilepsy. It reduces the severity of many severe to moderate diseases such as specific cancer types, Alzheimer's disease, type 2 diabetes, PCOS (polycystic ovary syndrome), obesity and epilepsy.

What is a Ketogenic diet? The diet, which is also known as the Keto diet, is a low-carb, high-fat diet and moderate-protein. It transforms the body into a state of ketosis. What is Ketosis? It is the body's metabolic process where it uses the stored fat for energy (fuel) when it is unable to get enough glucose (blood sugar). This forces the body to produce ketones that are used for fueling the body instead of glucose.

Though the Ketogenic diet is good for weight loss and has many other beneficial factors, it also comes with certain health issues and environmental concerns. The major environmental issue with all the meat-based diets begins with the most concerning issue – the source of these animal products (meat and dairy). Where do people source these animal-based food products? The bitter truth is, animals raised normally on CAFOs (controlled animal feeding operations) contribute to serious climate change and the worst part is the torture and abuse the poor animals have to go through. In addition to this, they affect the local environment and the animal-based products (meat/dairy) that come from these places are not nutritionally-dense but are nutritionally inferior.

Moreover, when you predominantly consume packaged meat such as hot dogs, salami, ham, sausages and bacon, you are consciously increasing the risk of type 2 diabetes, specific cancer types and heart disorders in your body. Formulating an eating plan that has a combination of both a vegetarian and ketogenic diet can work wonders if done in a proper manner. This is healthier and safer not just for you but also for the environment and the animals. Simply put, you get the benefits of both vegetarian and ketogenic diet in one dietary approach – the Vegetarian Ketogenic Diet.

The concept of this diet is low carb + high fat + moderate protein. Incorporating this in a well-balanced vegetarian diet can come in useful. Dairy and egg are equally cruel as meat products but since we are looking at a vegetarian keto diet, the book will be mentioning these products as meat alternatives. But if you are a vegan or would like to follow a plant-based diet, then you can always replace the eggs with vegan eggs or a flaxseed meal, and the dairy cheese and butter with vegan cheese and butter. There are plenty of vegan alternatives are available in the market.

Your body doesn't really need carbohydrates but the nutrients and fiber that comes from vegetables are important. Adding leafy vegetables to your diet can help you significantly, as they are rich in minerals, fiber and vitamins. Your carbs should come only from vegetables and it should be less than 20 grams to help maintain a healthy blood glucose level. Protein is another nutrient which is mandatory for your body for muscle mass. If you consume more protein, it gets converted into sugar just like how carbs get converted to glucose. Consuming too much protein might prevent your body from getting into the ketosis state. You feel satiated when you add more healthy fats to your food platter. It is essential to add fat in all the foods you consume to make sure you reach the required amount of fat that is needed daily.

If you have to adhere to the low-carb, high-fat keto diet perfectly, it is crucial to follow the following four suggestions:

- Make sure your carb consumption is only from low-carb veggies and your intake is less than or equal to 20 grams

- Ensure your fat consumption (at least 70 to 75 percent of calories) is from plant-based fats such as avocado oil, coconut oil, olive oil, etc

- Protein consumption should have only 20 to 25 percent calories which can be plant-based proteins such organic non-GMO tofu, peanuts, etc

- You can also use B12 and Iron supplements

In this book, we will be discussing the vegetarian keto diet and its possible role in weight loss. The chapters in this book will help you understand more about the ketogenic diet, its history, importance of a vegetarian keto diet, the health benefits and the do's and don'ts of the diet. This book also guides on how to start with the diet plan and has a few chapters dedicated to vegetarian-friendly keto diet recipes.

I hope this book serves as both an informative and interesting read to you!

Happy Reading!

Chapter One: Ketogenic Diet

Keto - the new buzzword is heating up the dietary debate in town but the fact is that the eating philosophy *Ketogenic Diet* isn't exactly new. It had, in fact, been used as an additional treatment approach for controlling epilepsy in the early 1920s. The *low-carb high-fat* diet came into the limelight again in the 1990s when a segment on ketosis was run by Dateline. They had highlighted the diet as a treatment option in the segment.

The surprise element here is - how did the keto diet go from epilepsy treatment to a weight-loss regime? If you are new to this dietary approach, then you need to know that more celebrities have showered praises on this eating pattern for its amazing weight-loss results. Celebs like Halle Berry, Vanessa Hudgens and Megan Fox had publicly endorsed this dietary approach, which made this a hot topic in various diet forums.

What exactly is a ketogenic diet? It is a dietary pattern where the consumption of low-carbohydrates and high fat in food forces your body to enter into a state of ketosis. During this ketosis process, instead of using carbs (glucose) as energy the body uses stored fat as energy.

When you follow the ketogenic diet, the fat you consume will give your body its daily dose of calories, which will approximately be around 60 to 80 percent. Your body will take close to 48 hours (maximum) or 24 hours (minimum) to start producing ketones when you continuously restrict carbs and eat more fat. These ketones are produced when your body decides to metabolize the stored fat for energy.

In a normal diet, carbohydrates become the primary source of energy for your body and therefore it metabolizes the consumed carbs (or stored glucose) as its fuel source. Most people get worried about the calorie-intake whenever they hear the term diet. But this is not the case with the ketogenic diet, as this dietary approach doesn't focus on specific calorie intake but rather the percentage of macronutrients.

Ketosis and Ketogenic Diet

A no-carb or extremely low-carb diet can force the body into the state of ketosis and this eating pattern is referred to as a ketogenic diet. When ketosis occurs, the molecules known as *ketones* get built up in the bloodstream.

Why does this happen? When the level of carbohydrate decreases in your body, it will cause the blood sugar levels to drop. The body will need fuel to continue to function normally and will force it to break down the stored fat (also known as calories) to use as its source of energy.

How is the keto diet responsible for this change? Since the keto diet involves low-carb consumption, the eating pattern forces a change in the body, i.e. the way the body converts its food to energy changes. When you eat less carbs and more fat, you force your body into a metabolic state wherein the body begins to burn the stored fat instead of carbohydrates for fuel. This metabolic state is referred to as ketosis. Because your body is not able to get enough glucose from the carbs you consume, the liver switches its usual approach by converting the fatty acids from your food or from your body (stored fat) into ketones. These ketones are the alternative energy source for the body to function normally.

This is where the health benefits begin – when your body burns ketones instead of glucose, it stimulates weight loss and reduces inflammation. As mentioned earlier, the ketogenic diet is nothing new as it has been in the system for close to a century. The original objective of the keto diet was to treat people with an epileptic condition. In the early 1920s, medical researchers found that the increased level of ketones in the blood reduced the epileptic seizures in the victims.

Even today, the ketogenic diet is used to treat children suffering from epilepsy if they don't respond well to the conventional anti-epileptic drugs.

How Does A Ketogenic Diet Work?

The keto diet converts your body into a fat-burning machine, which is the underlying reason for the weight-loss factor. When you follow a proper ketogenic diet, your body gets into a ketosis state that forces the body to burn fats for energy (fuel) instead of carbs. How exactly does this happen?

When you eat a meal that is rich in carbohydrates, your body will take the carbs from the food and convert them into glucose for energy. The insulin in your body will now move that glucose into your bloodstream. If the required carbohydrates are present in your body, then as expected the primary source of energy for your body becomes the alternative for glucose.

But things are not the same when you follow a ketogenic diet. Since the intake of carbohydrates is consistently kept low in a keto diet, your body will not be able to find enough carbs to convert them into glucose. Lack of carbs will force your body to look for an alternate source of energy to keep things going normally without any issues.

This is where the *fats* come into the picture. Due to the dearth of carbs in the body, the liver will take the fatty acids either from the stored fat or food consumed and convert them into ketones (also known as ketone bodies). These ketone bodies become the energy source instead of glucose and the process is referred to as ketosis (as mentioned earlier).

When the liver breaks down the fatty acids, three ketones are produced and they are,

- AcAc (Acetoacetate)

This ketone is the first created during the process of ketosis

- BHB (Beta-hydroxybutyric acid)

This ketone is formed from acetoacetate

- Acetone

This ketone is created instinctively as the by-product of acetoacetate

Benefits of A Ketogenic Diet

This popular dietary approach comes with a series of health benefits that include,

- Better sleep
- Satiety (Feels full even when the quantity is less)
- Better mood
- Healthy skin
- Clarity in thoughts (mental health)

Ketosis helps to burn fat which ultimately leads to considerable and rapid weight loss. The ketone bodies repress the hunger hormone (ghrelin) and amplify the cholecystokinin (CCK) – the one responsible in giving you that *satiated feel.* It is quite easy to go without eating for a longer period with reduced appetite in this dietary approach. This obviously motivates your body to look for the stored fats to fuel your system.

Another benefit of the keto diet is it increases your energy levels. This is because the body's metabolic state (ketosis) will help the brain to create more mitochondria. Mitochondria are the energy power generators within your body cells, i.e. more power in the cells will mean more energy to your body.

Following a keto diet will reduce inflammation, as this dietary approach is anti-inflammatory. This will help protect you against most of the degenerative illnesses such as cancer and Alzheimer's disease. A particular study had shown that it is possible to reduce the inflammation in the brain after an injury by following a keto diet.

Breakdown of Macronutrients

Who wouldn't love to eat a lot of fat? The ketogenic diet is all about eating loads of fat-based foods. But, you need to follow the breakdown percentage in the macronutrients when you eat a low or no carb, moderate protein and high fat diet.

The breakdown is as follows,

- Fat (70 to 80 percent)
- Protein (20 to 25 percent)
- Carbohydrates (5 to 10 percent)

If you are someone who has already been consuming fewer carbs, then you might have to eat even fewer dietary carbs to reach a healthy state of ketosis.

Ketosis is nothing artificial – you aren't forcing your body to do something that is unnatural. It is the natural function of the body. This body metabolism used to help our ancestors (cavemen) when they were devoid of food and were starving. When the cavemen couldn't find food for days, their body would naturally go for the stored fats and break them into ketones for the fuel source.

Similarly, when you are in keto, you are actually starving your body of carbs and in a way forcing (or conditioning) the body to turn to fat for energy. But you are not really starving!

You might experience certain side effects when you are altering your body to run on ketones for the first time. But when you continue with your diet as required, your body becomes adapted and begins to opt for fat as energy, thereby becoming a fat-burning machine.

Types of Ketogenic Diets

There are basically three types of ketogenic diets and they are,

- Standard Ketogenic Diet (SKD)
- Targeted Ketogenic Diet (TKD)
- Cyclic Ketogenic Diet (CKD)

And the last one that doesn't add on to the list is the restricted Ketogenic diet that is used for treatment and therapeutic purposes.

When you eat less than 50 gm net carbs in a day, you are following the *Standard Ketogenic diet.*

In the *Targeted Ketogenic diet*, you will consume extra carbohydrates an hour (or thirty minutes) before you do a high-intensity workout. Other than that, the eating pattern will be the same as that of a standard keto diet. Why do you need the extra carbs before exercising? Though there are no scientific evidences, it is believed that the glucose from the extra carbs can help boost the performance of your workout regimen.

In the *Cyclical Ketogenic diet*, you will have to eat a low carb diet that is less than 50 gm of net carbs in a day and high fat for five or six days in the week. The last day (7th day) will be the *carb re-feed* day where you will increase your carb-intake to roughly 150 gm.

When you cycle your carb intake in this manner, you tend to experience negative effects such as dry eyes, thyroid issues and fatigue, which usually happens to a few when long-term carb restriction happens.

Not everyone can manage with full ketosis! Adding carbs such as white rice, sweet potatoes and squash once a week will satisfy the need of carbs for the proper functioning of certain body systems.

How Will You Know If You Are In Ketosis?

You can check your ketone levels quite frequently to ensure your keto diet is working and your body is maintaining its ketosis state. The only way to check if your body has entered and is continuing to remain in ketosis is by testing the ketone levels. This is crucial to ensure you reap the entire benefits of the keto diet. When your body begins to burn the fat for energy and enters ketosis, the ketone bodies that are created will spill out into your breath, urine and blood.

When your ketone levels are at 0.8 (millimoles per liter), then your body has entered into ketosis. This can be tested and confirmed by using the blood meter, urine sticks or blood sticks. You can also use the breath analyzer to test the acetone levels in your breath.

Testing Ketone Levels In Urine

Urine strips will indicate the level of ketones in your body by color. The disadvantage of this method is that you cannot always rely on it – particularly when you have been in ketosis for quite some time.

Sometimes, the reading might show lower ketone levels even if your body is burning them because your body is more efficient in using the ketones. You might also get inconsistent readings if your electrolyte levels are high. Hydration in your body can also affect the reading.

Testing Ketone Levels In Breath

You can use the breath meter to test the acetone level (the ketone that shows up) on your breath. Like urine testing, this cannot be considered as your only method for testing as the discrepancy in reading might occur if you have a cold or thyroid issues.

Testing Ketone Levels In The Blood

The accurate way to check and monitor the ketone levels is through blood testing. You can use a blood strip or blood glucose meter to check the ketone levels in your blood. But this is a bit costly compared to the other two methods.

However, you can also check if your body has gone into the ketosis stage by simply tracking the way your body feels. A few signs are:

- You don't feel as hungry as before because the ketone bodies repress your hunger hormones making you feel satiated for a longer time
- Few people experience a weird metallic taste in their mouth when the ketone levels increase
- If you are losing weight, voila, you are in ketosis as the process burns the stored fat

How Do You Start A Ketogenic Diet?

You can start a keto diet by following the six steps mentioned below:

- Decide and finalize
- Check your ideal weight
- Calculate the macronutrients
- Shop and stock the required food items
- Eliminate the carbs from your diet
- Include proteins, greens and fat to your diet

Once you have made your decision and finalized on it, you need to get started with the new Ketogenic lifestyle.

But before you get into it, two crucial steps that need to be followed are *checking your ideal weight and calculating the macronutrients you need to consume.*

What do you mean by an ideal body weight? It is the body weight that is apt for your age, gender and height. The main factor when it comes to ideal body weight is *height* – followed by the *gender* and the *age*. Humans cannot grow after a certain age because of which height is considered as an important factor in finding one's ideal weight. You can calculate your ideal weight using the weight calculator at

https://www.calculator.net/ideal-weight-calculator.html

For instance, a woman who currently weighs around 160 pounds with a height of 5'3" should ideally weigh 116 pounds. For her to attain the ideal weight, she will need to know how much food she needs to eat. And this can be achieved by calculating the macronutrients.

What are macronutrients? Nutrients are substances that are required for metabolism, growth and other functionalities of the body. Your body requires certain nutrients in large amounts and these nutrients are referred to as macronutrients. Humans usually need three important macronutrients,

- Carbohydrates
- Protein
- Fats

Each of these macronutrients provides energy to the body in the form of calories. Calculating these macronutrients will help start a proper ketogenic diet plan.

Chapter Two: Vegetarian Ketogenic Diet

Most people remove meat from their diet for the environment or for the sake of animals, as they prefer to have a cruelty-free diet. But there are a few others who choose a vegetarian diet, as they believe it is a much healthier option compared to the meat-eating routine. Vegetarian diets are usually rich in nutrients and carbohydrates as they come with loads of legumes, starchy vegetables and grains. But this form of diet might not suit people who are affected by diabetes – especially if they are looking to control their blood sugar levels without medication. The other issue with a high-carb, low-fat vegetarian eating routine is most people constantly feel hungry – they never feel satiated.

The idea of a Vegetarian Ketogenic diet may come as a blessing to all those individuals who would like to avoid meat but still reap the benefits of a ketogenic lifestyle. How will you define a vegetarian ketogenic diet? A diet that restricts the intake of carbohydrates and is free of poultry, meat and fish can be referred to as the keto-vegetarian or vegetarian ketogenic diet. You gain the benefits of a ketogenic diet and also reduce your carbon footprint, improve your health and decrease the abuse of animals.

How do you implement the keto-vegetarian diet? Are there any particular rules to be followed? Yes, there are few rules that you have to keep in mind:

- Do away with all forms of animal flesh (meat, fowl flesh and fish) from your food platter.

- Ensure the total carb consumption for the day to be equal to or less than 35 gm.

- Minimum 70 percent of your calories should come from the fat you consume.

- Eat a lot of low-carb vegetables.

- If you don't get enough nutrients such as zinc, iron and vitamins (DHA, D3, EPA) from your food, use supplements or fortified food items.

- Let 35 percent of your calories be from dairy (or vegan alternatives) and plant-based proteins.

- Check your macronutrient needs and calories using the keto calculator before you proceed with your diet chart (https://www.ruled.me/keto-calculator/)

Different Types of Vegetarians

Vegetarians are usually thought of as people who quit meat products but the different categories of vegetarians mentioned below will tell you otherwise. It has been categorized in order of the most liberal to the strictest:

- *Pescatarians*

They consume eggs, seafood and dairy but completely avoid red meat and fowl flesh. This eating routine is referred to as semi-vegetarian and isn't much riskier in terms of nutrient deficiencies when compared to the people who include meat into their diet.

- *Lacto-ovo vegetarians*

They consume eggs and dairy but completely avoid meat, seafood and poultry. This form of vegetarian diet is quite common in Europe, the United States and other western countries.

- *Lacto vegetarians*

They consume dairy but strictly avoid meat, eggs, fowl flesh and seafood. This form of vegetarian diet is followed in India.

- *Vegans*

They basically avoid anything coming from animals – dairy, seafood, meat, eggs, poultry and any form of animal products that include honey. These people refuse not only to consume but also to use any products made from animals (flesh, skin or any of their body parts). They don't encourage industries that breed or misuse or harass animals (factory farming, backyard breeding, entertainment such as circus, zoos, etc.)

It is possible to incorporate the ketogenic diet to most of these vegetarian categories but the most liberal forms of the vegetarian diet will let a wide range of food choices to the ones who follow them. For instance, a vegan keto diet will have a lot more restrictions when compared to a Lacto-Ovo vegetarian keto diet.

Protein is the only essential nutrient that cannot be made by the body and has to be acquired only through food. When you consume a proper and complete protein diet, you get to obtain all the nine essential amino acids. It is believed that plants contain only some of these essential amino acids while animal protein provides all of them.

This is because different plant-based foods contain different types of amino acids. So, as a vegan, when you exclude all forms of animal products, you completely rely on a combination of seeds, grains and legumes to get all the essential amino acids your body will need (it isn't impossible but will need dedicated attention to details). Unfortunately, many of these plant foods that have a good amount of protein are high on carbs. Therefore, they cannot be added to the keto diet as the diet restricts carbs to only 20 grams of net carbs (i.e. net carbs = total carbs – fiber).

However, it is still possible to go on a low-carb diet for people who want to completely eliminate all forms of animal products from their diet. The low carb, vegan and non-keto diet is called as the *Eco-Atkins diet*. This low-carb diet is completely plant-based. Why isn't this diet considered a keto diet if it is a low-carb diet? Though the diet has fewer carbs, it includes grains that yield 60 grams or more of the net carbs in a day.

Vegetarians and Carbs

Vegetarians, much like the non-vegetarians, also have problems with their body weight. It is no news that they will have to seriously modify their diets to deal with their weight as a classic vegetarian diet has less fat and more carbs. Few vegetarians have difficulty in processing their carbs, which ultimately leads to weight gain and various other health issues.

What is the difference between good carbs and bad carbs?

When it comes to losing weight, the only thing that is taken into consideration seriously on a ketogenic diet is your consumption of the amount of carbs. But as a vegetarian, if you are looking for overall health and wellness, then it is crucial for you to understand the difference between good carbs and bad carbs.

Good carbs are foods that are not processed or minimally processed. These food items are rich in nutrients and high on fiber content.

Bad carbs are heavily processed foods that are extremely high on carbohydrates. When you consume these heavily processed high-carb foods, they enter your bloodstream much faster than the good carbs as they get converted to sugar (glucose) more rapidly.

Why are bad carbs not good for your overall health and wellness?

Carbs, in general, raise your blood sugar levels but these heavily processed bad carbs are quickly absorbed by your body and processed much faster than the good carbs. The good carbs that are close to their natural state is mostly rich in nutrients and fiber. The natural process that happens after consuming the carbs is:

- Carbs are converted into sugar (which is also referred to as glucose)

- This glucose is then released into your bloodstream where it is used as the energy source (fuel).

- This causes the blood sugar levels to rise in your body, which ultimately gives you the required energy.

- Your pancreas will release insulin to help these glucose contents (sugar) to be used by your bodies.

- This release of insulin allows your body to process the sugar of the carbs as fuel.

The problem arises only when you consume too many carbs as they will be responsible for your blood sugar levels to shoot up. This causes the corresponding insulin, which was released to block your body's ability to use this increased glucose as fuel. This will result in it getting stored as calories that ultimately cause the weight gain.

It doesn't stop here – the issue turns into a nasty cycle where your blood sugar levels increase rapidly and then again decreases quickly. When this cycle continues, your energy levels go down making it hard for you to focus. This rapid fall in energy can cause hunger issues in many which ultimately leads to the need for increasing the blood sugars. Naturally, you will consume more carbs to survive throughout the day as you are in dire need of energy and the hunger pangs are already frustrating you.

How do you limit your carb-intake?

The most common mistake that vegetarians tend to make when they follow a ketogenic diet is that they unknowingly eat too many carbs. Why does this happen? It is because most of the favorite food items of vegetarians are heavily loaded with carbohydrates. A few of them include:

- Fruit (bananas, apples, oranges, etc)

- Legumes (Peas, Lentils, black beans, etc)

- Tubers (Yams, Potatoes, etc)

- Grains (Corn, Cereal, Wheat, rice, etc)

- Sugar (Maple syrup, honey, agave, etc)

All of the foods mentioned above are so high in carbs that one serving can cross the actual carb limit for the day. Just because you cannot have these high-carb foods, doesn't mean you need to worry about your keto-friendly low carb food option. You are not going to get stuck with lettuce and eggs.

You still have the following food options that you can eat without any guilt:

- Low-carb sweeteners (Monk fruit, erythritol, stevia and other options)

- Leafy greens (Kale, Spinach, etc)

- Seeds and nuts (Almonds, pumpkin seeds, pistachios, sunflower seeds, etc)

- Vegan meat options (low-carb vegan meats, seitan, tempeh, tofu and other plant-based high protein food)

- Above the ground vegetables (zucchini, broccoli, cauliflower, etc)

- Other fats (MCT oil, coconut oil, olive oil, etc)

- Avocado and berries such as blackberries, raspberries, blueberries and other low-glycemic impact berries)

- Eggs and high-fat dairy (butter, hard cheeses, high fat cream, etc)

Bad carbs that need to be eliminated from your diet

You will need to make sure you do away with all those high-carb heavily processed foods such as white flour, white sugar, etc. These carb-laden foods are full of bad carbs, which are not good for your health and are completely non-keto. Other foods include:

- Pretzels
- Tortillas
- Fruit juices
- Non-diet sodas and carbonated sugar-rich drinks
- White bread
- White Pasta
- Crackers
- Chips
- Carrots, Sweet Potatoes, Potatoes, Corn and yams
- Low-fiber cereals which have sugar content in it
- White rice

Keto-Friendly Vegetarian Fats

High-fat dairy and eggs will always find a significant place in most part of your keto meals. But it is not going to be your only source of fat. The interesting fact here is you can replace all the animal fats that you frequently use in baking and cooking with various plant-based oils.

Check out the list of plant-based oils given below along with their uses,

- *MCT Oil*

This oil is usually derived from palm oil and coconut oil. It contains saturated fatty acids such as medium-chain triglycerides that go directly into the liver when consumed. These fatty acids skip the normal routine of fat digestion and go straight into the liver where they get broken down into ketones for fuel. You can add this oil to almost all your food items such as sauces, fat bombs, salad dressings, hot drinks (tea, coffee) and smoothies. They help you boost your potent energy levels.

- *Avocado Oil*

This oil has tons of healthy mono-unsaturated fats that can be used for cooking, deep-frying and baking. The oil has the highest smoke point of 520 degrees

Fahrenheit when compared to the other cooking oils making it the perfect cooking and baking oil.

- *Olive Oil*

It is one of the healthiest oils that you can consume. Ensure you use the oil to increase the fat content of all your vegetarian keto meals. Adding this oil also enhances the flavor of the spices and contents in the meal. The oil can become unhealthy when it oxidizes, so ensure you don't cook with the oil at a temperature that is anywhere below 405 degrees Fahrenheit.

- *Coconut oil*

This oil contains an abundant quantity of fatty acids that can serve as the ideal source of fuel for people who follow a ketogenic diet. Using this oil for baking, making desserts, fat bombs and cooking enrich the nutrient content of the meal. Like butter, this oil needs to be cooked or baked under 350 degrees Fahrenheit.

- *Red Palm Oil*

This oil can double up as a vitamin supplement as it is rich in Vitamin E and Vitamin A. The oil has a rich buttery texture with a mild flavor that tastes like carrots. Using this oil in cooking can enhance the flavor of seeds, vegan meat and nuts.

Though there are plenty of plant-based oils that you can consume, the oils mentioned above are the most resourceful and healthiest of the lot. However, there is no hard-and-fast rule that your fat consumption should be only from these oils. You can also go ahead and get some extra fat for your body along with essential minerals and vitamins by including the following fatty foods to your keto-vegetarian meals,

- Avocado is not only rich in fats but is also packed with minerals, vitamins and antioxidants whereas avocado oil concentrates only on the fat part of the macros.
- The healthy fat-rich addition to your diet that you shouldn't be avoiding are nuts. Cashews and macadamia nuts are filled with healthy

mono-unsaturated fats with the lowest amount of inflammatory omega 6 fats. But before you add them to your diet ensure you know the number of carbs these nuts hold. Sometimes you may come out of ketosis by eating too many cashews.

- Another healthy fat addition to your vegetarian keto diet is seeds such as flaxseeds, pumpkin seeds, sunflower seeds and sesame seeds. But you cannot rely on them entirely as a stable dietary fat food as they contain high levels of inflammatory omega-6 fats.

When you combine these fat-packed plant foods and plant-based oils, you wouldn't even need to add high-fat dairy and eggs to your vegetarian keto diet to achieve your fat needs.

Keto-friendly Sources of Vegetarian Protein

Though meat is one of the richest sources of protein, you don't necessarily need them to meet your protein requirements if you eat cheese and eggs regularly. However, even if you are an ardent lover of cheese and a super cool chef who can prepare delicious egg-cheese meals, eating them almost regularly may cause other health issues.

It is therefore advisable to consume the following protein sources to achieve your protein needs,

Tofu

Tofu, which is made from soybeans, is a well-known alternative for cottage cheese (known as paneer in India). It is high in calcium and protein. Using it in your meals can work as a realistic delicious substitute for fish, meat and poultry. Tofu is usually mushy and soft but if you are using it as a meat-alternative in any of your recipes, then you can go for extra-firm tofu. It will be chewy and firm. Ensure you marinate the extra-firm tofu with the required seasoning or flavors for it to absorb all the flavors before you cook.

Tempeh

This fermented form of soy is much firmer than tofu and has a grainy texture. It can be an awesome substitute for beef and fish. How do you use this fermented soy form in your food? All you have to do is grind it up in a food processor, slice it or dice it. If the tempeh is a little bitter, then just steam it for a few minutes before you use it.

Since both tempeh and tofu is made from soy, you will need to take note of how you feel after you consume them. Though soy is healthy for many people, some will face certain health issues as it contains a plant compound known as the goitrogen. This might impair the functionality of the thyroid glands.

In case you feel any of the following symptoms as a result of your increased intake of soy-based products, then you will have to limit the amount of soy products you consume.

- Dry skin
- Fatigue
- Constipation
- Unexplained weight gain
- Sensitivity to cold

You might also have to supplement your diet with foods that are rich in iodine in such cases.

To avoid these issues, make sure you get soy products that are 100 percent organic. So, the tofu and tempeh you purchase should be made from organic soy. The usual soy products normally contain traces of dangerous chemicals such as herbicides, pesticides that are sprayed in huge amounts on those GMO soybeans

Seitan

It is a vegetarian meat substitute that is also referred to as wheat meat. Seitan is made from tamari (or soy sauce), wheat gluten, garlic, seaweed and ginger. This vegan meat is an excellent source of iron – it is low in fat and high in protein.

But if you are gluten-sensitive, it is best to avoid seitan as it is mainly made from gluten protein and therefore will contain loads of gluten.

Seeds and Nuts

Most of the nuts and seeds are richly packed with protein and fat. The following seeds and nuts contain the most protein (per 100 gm of the seeds/nuts),

- Almonds (21 gm)
- Flaxseed (18 gm)
- Pumpkin seeds (30 gm)
- Sunflower seeds (19 gm)

- Pistachios (21 gm)

But when you add these seeds and nuts to your food also keep a note of their carb contents (per 100 gm of the seeds/nuts) too,

- Almonds (22 gm of total carbs)
- Flaxseed (19 gm)
- Pumpkin seeds (54 gm)
- Sunflower seeds (20 gm)
- Pistachios (28 gm)

How is it possible to forget about the peanuts when you talk about protein? Though you cannot place it under the nuts or seeds category, as it is technically a legume, peanut is a rich source of protein with low carbs. Peanuts are low in carbs (16 gm of total carbs in every 100 gm of peanuts) and are high in protein (approximately 24 gm in every 100 gm of peanuts.)

The Other Alternatives

You have a lot of keto-friendly vegetarian and vegan alternatives when you cut down your egg and cheese consumption. Few of the options are:

- Use coconut cream instead of heavy dairy cream

- Use coconut oil or non-dairy butter instead of dairy butter

- Use non-dairy cheese instead of dairy cheese

- Use non-dairy based soft cheese instead of dairy cream cheese

- Use nut-based yogurt or coconut yogurt instead of dairy yogurt and sour cream

- Use Vegan Egg or The Vegg or Flaxseed meal instead of eggs

Whenever you opt for keto-friendly vegan or vegetarian options, ensure you check for any hidden carbs, added sugars or hydrogenated oils. Don't forget to check for the percentage of the protein and fat content.

Chapter Three: How To Get Started?

One of the most sustainable diets for your health, the environment and for the animals is now combined with a ketogenic diet – *the vegetarian ketogenic diet.* Now, that you have understood the difference between the conventional keto diet and vegetarian keto diet, it is time to get started.

Action Plan

To get started with a veg-friendly keto diet, you will need to make sure you follow the simple steps mentioned below,

- Carb-restriction
- Including high-quality protein
- Eat vegetables (at least one to three servings) twice a day

- Use plant-based healthy fat oils for salad dressings and cooking
- Seasoning food with different spices and herbs

Carb-restriction

It is crucial to limit your intake of net carbs to 20 gm per day so that your body enters the ketosis state and remains in the state until your diet cycle completes. You will need to avoid legumes, quinoa, pulses and buckwheat even though they are rich protein sources as they are too high in carbs. Adding this to your diet will hinder your keto routine. Ensure you stay away from starchy vegetables, low-fat dairy products, high-sugar content fruit, certain berries and milk.

Including high-quality protein

It is essential to add a high-quality source of protein to every single meal you have. Your quality of protein in a vegetarian diet will improve when you combine eggs and dairy with low-carb keto-friendly plant proteins such as seeds and nuts. On an average, people who follow a keto diet will need somewhere between 60 and 100 grams of protein in a day. This also depends on their age, weight, activity level and body composition.

The energy levels are much better when you eat around 1 to 1.6 gm of protein per kilogram of your body weight. The top three sources of protein are:

- *Egg*

It has an easily digestible high-quality protein that provides choline (linked to the better functioning of the brain). Two large eggs contain 1 gm carb and 14 gm protein.

- *Hemp Seeds*

These seeds are rich in soluble fiber and are a great source of potassium, magnesium and omega-3 fatty acids. It is extremely high in protein content. 1 ounce of hemp seeds contains 1 gm net carb and 9 gm protein.

- *Greek yogurt*

It is an excellent source of magnesium, calcium and potassium; it also provides the probiotics that are extremely beneficial for immunity and gut health. It is considered to be rich in high-quality protein. 6 ounces of Greek Yogurt contains 5 to 7 gm carbs and 15 to 20 gm protein.

In addition to these three protein sources, there are several other vegetarian keto protein sources such as:

- *Semi-hard and hard cheese* (gouda, Swiss, provolone, cheddar, etc)

One ounce of the cheese contains 0 to 1 gm carb and 7 to 8 gm protein

- *Almond or Peanut butter* (2 tablespoons of the butter contains 4 gm net carbs and 7 to 8 gm protein)
- *Cottage cheese* (6 ounces contain 6 gm carbs and 20 gm protein)

- *Soft Cheese* (Feta, Queso Blanco, Brie, Blue cheese, Camembert, etc)

1 ounce contains o to 1 gm carb and 4 to 6 gm protein

- *Romano and Parmesan cheese* (1 ounce contains 1 gm carb and 9 to 10 gm protein)

Apart from these, you will also get a minimum 2 gm of protein per cup from most vegetables. Avoid going for protein bars, protein powders or protein shakes and try to get maximum protein from the real, natural food.

Eat vegetables (at least one to three servings) twice a day

There are plenty of vegetables that are completely keto-friendly and the best part is most of these vegetables taste delicious and are rich in nutrients. They give you the required dose of fiber and also meet your micro and macronutrient needs.

The top five vegetables that are keto-friendly are:

- Cauliflower (rich in fiber and vitamin C, perfect keto-friendly substitute for rice and mashed potatoes. 1 serving = 4 gm net carbs)
- Avocado (Though it is technically a fruit, it can be used as a vegetable substitute. Rich in fiber, potassium and magnesium. 1 serving = 2 gm net carb)
- Spinach (rich in magnesium, iron and potassium. 1 serving = 1 gm net carb)
- Brussels Sprouts (rich in folate, vitamin C and potassium. 1 serving = 5 gm net carb)
- Zucchini (rich in potassium, vitamin C and vitamin B6. Perfect substitute for noodles. 1 serving = 3 gm net carb)

Use plant-based healthy fat oils for salad dressings and cooking

Consuming healthy fats makes you feel satiated and you don't feel as hungry for longer hours. Adding healthy fats to your recipes improves the texture of the food and makes it taste delicious. These fats also play a major role in absorbing the fat-soluble vitamins such as vitamin D, K, E and A.

It is important to choose the healthiest types of fats as most of your calories are obtained from fats in a ketogenic diet. Though seed oils and vegetable oils such as safflower, canola, corn and sunflower are rich in fats, they have been associated with inflammation and are highly processed.

It is advisable to choose healthy condiments and keto fats such as coconut oil, avocado oil, olive oil, ghee and butter both for cooking and dressing.

Seasoning the food with different spices and herbs

It is quite easy to try different varieties of recipes for a vegetarian diet if you add more spices and herbs to your cooking routine. The additional advantage is that they come with numerous sources of micronutrients and are pretty low in net carbs. Experiment your recipes with rosemary, basil, cinnamon and few other spices or herbs which you have never tried. Who knows, you might even find your new favorites!

Must-haves (Vegetables, Condiments, Fruit and Spices)

The major thing you need to keep note of while following a ketogenic diet is to make sure to keep your fat content high. In addition to this, you will also have to include healthy low-carb vegetables, which can provide more fiber and nutrients. You will need to get enough to eat and also feel satiated at the same time. Don't restrict yourself from trying new vegetables. Explore and prepare veggies in different ways. If you are not too keen with raw salads, dry roast, bake or boil the vegetables. Add a lot of herbs and spices as seasonings. You can also cook them with coconut oil or butter to enjoy a delicious salad.

The following are some of the must-have vegetarian foods that are completely keto-friendly:

Low-carb vegetables

- Kale
- Swiss Chard
- Asparagus
- Broccoli
- Winter and Summer Squash
- Cauliflower
- Onions
- Tomatoes
- Garlic
- Spinach
- Collard Greens
- Lettuce
- Green beans
- Cucumber
- Red and white cabbage
- Bell peppers
- Mushrooms
- Eggplants

Condiments

The best choice is to make all your condiments at home but if it is difficult, you can go ahead and buy the following as they have no carbs or fewer carbs (microscopic quantity).

- Worcestershire sauce
- Yellow mustard
- Ketchup (Sugar-free)
- High-fat Salad dressings (Low sugar or sugar-free)
- Coconut aminos
- Soy sauce
- Hot sauces
- Mayonnaise (made with cage-free eggs)
- Sugar-free Sauerkraut

Fruit

Keto diets restrict almost all type of fruit but you can still have certain fruit or berries that have low-carbs and low-sugar. If you are having these fruits, you need to have them only at the end of the day before you go to sleep.

-   Strawberries
-   Blueberries
-   Blackberries
-   Raspberries

Spices

-   Oregano
-   Rosemary
-   Cilantro
-   Chili powder
-   Cinnamon
-   Lime or lemon juices

- Basil

- Parsley

- Thyme

- Cayenne pepper

- Cumin

- Nutmeg

- Pepper

- Salt

Though there are different types of keto diets, the strictest versions of the diet will limit your intake of carbohydrates to nothing more than 20 gm in a day. If you are looking for an effective and faster weight-loss regimen, then it is important to follow lower-carb diets. However, not many people can stay on such low-carb diets for a long term.

The best way to stick to the ketogenic diet is to follow a moderate keto diet that not only helps you to maintain or lose weight but also keeps you healthy. You can follow the guidelines mentioned below for better results:

-   1400 to 1500 (daily calorie count)

-   25 to 35 gm (daily fiber intake)

-   Equal to or less than 50 gm (daily carb intake)

-   50 to 60 gm (daily fat intake)

Meal Ideas for a Vegetarian Ketogenic Diet

These are just sample meal ideas for a vegetarian version of Keto diet. You can tweak it according to your taste and ideas but ensure you stick to the macronutrient levels.

Breakfast

-   Eggs and Vegetables with avocado (fried in olive oil or coconut oil)

-   Eggs frittata with avocado and asparagus

-   Vegetable and feta omelet (fried in olive oil or coconut oil)

- Full-fat smoothie (made from full-fat yogurt, stevia extract, few berries, ice, almond butter and coconut cream)

Lunch

- Avocado and Egg salad
- Mixed greens salad with mozzarella, olives, onions, lemon juice, avocado, pesto, bell pepper, a couple of nuts and extra-virgin olive oil dressing
- Low-carb vegetarian Greek salad with fresh Greek spices, tomatoes, olives, feta, onions and extra-virgin olive oil dressing
- Stir-fried cauliflower rice with eggs and vegetables

Dinner

- Cauliflower crusted cheese pizza with broccoli
- Zucchini-noodle pasta and keto alfredo sauce
- Portobello steak with kale salad and cauliflower mashed potatoes
- Coconut oil-fried eggplant parmesan

Chapter Four: Tips and Guidelines

It is important to be familiar with the right portion sizes of the food you eat – especially when you are following a specific dietary approach. The Mayo Clinic has come up with interesting visual reminders for you to stay on track.

- Your fruit serving shouldn't be any larger than the size of a tennis ball

- One serving of different vegetables (put together) shouldn't exceed the size of a baseball

- The dairy serving should only be the size of three or four dice put together.

- One serving of carbs should not exceed the size of a hockey puck.

- One single serving of fat shouldn't be anything larger than two dice put together.

- Your protein serving should be the size of a deck of cards

Never be afraid to experiment when it comes to choosing your food. Be open to new foods and find interesting ways of preparing your old favorites or traditional dishes. Add more spices to your food and don't fail to try new spices – especially the ones you have never tried or heard off. It will be fun!

When you find new and appetizing ways to prepare your dishes, you tend to be consistent with your eating pattern. Maintaining a nutritious and healthy way of eating will always be beneficial for you on a long-term basis.

The Do's and Don'ts of KETO

Irrespective of you being new to keto or not, you may end up making some mistakes which can lead you to come to a state of a standstill as you aren't getting the required results you ought to be getting. Sometimes, you may also face disturbances in your overall health condition.

Most people start a ketogenic diet to handle their weight problems but there are also a few of them who look at this diet as a therapy. They might want to stop their medication for high blood pressure or Type 2 diabetes. There are some who follow the keto diet to maintain their health and overall wellness. Some would choose the diet to stay strong and energized all through the day.

Do's of KETO

- Eat real food. Avoid packaged or chemical-infused food products. Go for organic vegetables and fruit.

- Replace your electrolytes with vegetable broth instead of your sugar-filled energy drinks or diet Gatorade. Ensure your body gets minimum 2 teaspoons of salt in a day.

- Eat only healthy fats – plenty of them! Include MCT oil, olive oil, avocado oil, coconut oil, heavy cream, extra-virgin plant-based oils. Fat is a brain food – it gives mental clarity and is an excellent source of energy

-   Use only natural sweeteners (alternative for sugar) such as stevia, erythritol, etc

Don'ts of KETO

-   Don't eat so-called sugar-free candies, low-carb tortillas, low-carb bars, diet soda, shakes, frozen meals (that can be heated and consumed), zero-calorie artificial-sweetened drinks or any form of low-carb packaged ready-to-eat products.

-   Don't eat so-called low-fat or fat-free yogurt or cheese. STRICTLY NO! You will need to eat plenty of healthy fats and full-fat cheese. For a keto diet, you need to have full-fat yogurt and full-fat cream. You see low fat or no-fat in the label, turn around and walk away!

- Avoid eating bad fats – hydrogenated oil, corn oil, soybean oil, canola oil and vegetable oil.

- Eliminate fast food from your diet chart. It is loaded with preservatives and chemicals. They don't use real food ingredients anymore – salads have hidden sugars, cheese is no longer real organic cheese, and the fries are full of preservatives. No more McDonald's or Pizza Huts or Burger King.

- Don't look at the nutritional details after you have consumed the respective food item. Always look for the nutritional breakup before you eat, not after you eat!

Ways To Avoid Nutrient Deficiencies On A Keto-Vegetarian Diet

Most vegetarians rely heavily on legumes and grains to achieve their daily dosage of micronutrients. But when the keto diet restricts these foods because of their high carb content, then it is crucial to ensure you consume all the required quantities of the following nutrients:

- Potassium

- Vitamin D

- Calcium

- Omega-3 fatty acids

- Magnesium

- Zinc

- Vitamin B12

You need to make sure you are consuming loads of lower-carb vegetables and high-quality vegetarian protein sources. This will help manage your intake of the micronutrients on a vegetarian ketogenic diet.

To make sure your body gets the required range of micronutrients, make sure you eat the following nutrient-rich foods on a daily basis. This will help you avoid the risk of a nutrient-deficiency.

Vegetables

- Broccoli
- Kale
- Spinach
- Artichokes
- Brussels Sprouts
- Mushrooms
- Swiss Chard

Fruit

- Olives
- Avocado

Dairy

- Cheese
- Plain Greek Yogurt

Seeds and Nuts

- Chia seeds
- Hemp seeds
- Pumpkin seeds

- Flax seeds

- Walnuts

- Almonds

Others

- Cocoa (unsweetened)

- 100 percent dark chocolate

If you don't feel at your best even after eating all these nutrient-dense foods, then you might have to pay attention to the nutrients you are specifically deficient in. On the contrary, you don't particularly need to worry about micronutrients if you are regularly consuming a wide range of nutrient-rich foods. *Make it simple; simple does the trick!*

It is definitely possible to be both vegetarian and keto. You need to choose the right food that is rich in the key nutrients, experiment with different protein and vegetable combinations and use a wide range of spices and herbs. Let your keto-vegetarian lifestyle be satisfying, healthy and sustainable.

Vegetarian Keto Shopping List

Now that you are aware of the food items you can include in your regular diet to force your body to enter into ketosis, it is time to make the shopping list and ensure your kitchen is packed with necessary vegetables, fruit, nuts, spices, seeds and other condiments.

Take a trip to your nearby grocery store and get the following vegetarian ketogenic food list based on your weekly meal plan.

Non-Starchy Vegetables

- Asparagus
- Cauliflower
- Celery
- Mushrooms
- Tomatoes
- Leafy Greens
- Carrots

- Onions

- Eggplant

- Peppers

- Turnips

- Brussels Sprouts

- Artichokes

- Beets

- Cucumbers

Fruit with low-sugar content

- Strawberries

- Cherries

- Blackberries

- Raspberries

- Plums

- Apples

- Oranges

Healthy Fats

-   Nuts

-   Coconut oil

-   Olive oil

-   Grass-fed butter

-   Avocados

-   Seeds

-   MCT oil

-   Palm oil

-   Ghee

Vegetarian Protein

-   Tempeh

-   Seeds

-   Nutritional yeast

-   Eggs

-   Nuts

-   Spirulina

-   Natto

Precautionary Measures To Be Taken On Keto-Veg Diet

The keto diet is basically a high-fat diet but the crucial factor here is you need to be wise while choosing the types of fat that needs to be included in your diet. It is necessary to consume healthy fats. You may achieve your regular dosage of fat intake by piling your plate with highly processed faux meat but the downside is, you wipe out the prospective health-promoting properties the keto diet can give you.

It is true that a plant-based keto diet or a vegetarian keto diet comes with a whole host of health benefits but you may increase the risk of nutritional deficiencies if you follow a poorly planned vegan or vegetarian keto diet. You will have to add a good variety of nutrient-dense foods along with your plant-based protein food items.

Make sure you include healthy fats, low-sugar fruit, seeds, fermented foods, nuts and non-starchy vegetables as your stable food items on a regular basis. The more nutritious your food is, the lesser your risk is of getting a nutrient-deficit.

In case you have any doubts or queries, it is best to consult with a dietician or doctor to find out what might work best for you.

The upcoming chapters will have a few easy vegetarian keto recipes to help you with a complete meal plan.

Chapter Five: Vegetarian Keto Breakfast Recipes

Keto Zucchini Bread with Walnuts

Servings: 16

Ingredients:

- 3 eggs (large ones)
- 1 cup organic zucchini (grated)
- 2 1/2 cups almond flour
- 1/2 cup walnuts (chopped)
- 1 1/2 cups erythritol
- 1 teaspoon cinnamon (ground)
- 1 teaspoon vanilla extract
- 1/4 teaspoon ginger (ground)
- 1 1/2 teaspoons baking powder
- 1/2 teaspoon nutmeg
- 1/2 cup olive oil
- 1/2 teaspoon salt
- Nonstick cooking spray

Method:

1. Preheat oven to 350 degrees Fahrenheit.

2. Take a small bowl and crack the eggs.

3. Whisk together the oil, vanilla extract and the eggs. Set aside.

4. Mix the baking powder, salt, ginger, cinnamon, almond flour, erythritol and nutmeg together in another bowl.

5. Squeeze out the excess water from the zucchini using cheesecloth or a paper towel.

6. Add the zucchini to the egg mixture and whisk together until well-combined.

7. Add the almond flour mixture to the zucchini-egg mixture slowly.

8. Use a hand mixer and blend the contents thoroughly until smooth and well blended.

9. Grease a 9x5 loaf pan with nonstick cooking spray and transfer the zucchini flour mixture.

10.   Spread evenly and sprinkle the chopped walnuts over the mixture. Press the walnuts into the batter using the backside of a spoon or spatula.

11.   Bake for 70 minutes until the walnuts are browned and the bread mixture is set.

12.   Transfer to a plate and serve!

Low-carb Cauliflower Hash Browns

Servings: 4

Ingredients:

- 15 ounces cauliflower (rinsed, trimmed and grated)
- 1/2 yellow onion (grated)
- 4 ounces butter or 8 tablespoons melted coconut oil
- 3 eggs
- 2 pinches pepper
- 1 teaspoon salt

Method:

1. Take a large bowl and place the grated cauliflower in it.

2. Add the onion, salt, pepper and crack the eggs into the bowl.

3. Mix the contents well until blended thoroughly.

4. Heat 3 tablespoons of coconut oil in a large skillet over medium heat.

5. Spoon the cauliflower batter and place the scoops in the hot oil. Flatten them to 3 inches in diameter carefully.

6. You should be able to fry 3 hash browns in one go.

7. Let it fry for 5 minutes on each side and carefully flip it to the other side. Allow it to fry for another 5 minutes.

8. You will need to adjust the heat to ensure the hashes don't get burnt.

9. Be careful while flipping the hashes as it might fall apart if you do it too soon. Let the edges turn crispy and sport a golden brown color.

10. Transfer to a plate and repeat steps 5 to 9 with the remaining batter. Add more oil if needed.

11. Serve warm and enjoy!

Keto Coconut Porridge

Servings: 1

Ingredients:

- 4 tablespoons + extra coconut cream
- 1 egg
- 1 tablespoon coconut flour
- 1 pinch psyllium husk powder (ground)
- 2 tablespoons butter or coconut oil
- 1 pinch salt
- Fresh or frozen berries (for garnishing)

Method:

1. Heat the coconut oil over medium-high heat in a non-stick saucepan.

2. Reduce the heat to low when the oil melts and crack the egg into it.

3. Add the coconut cream, coconut flour, psyllium husk powder and salt to the egg in the pan.

4. Mix well until the contents are completely incorporated.

5. Let it cook for 10 minutes as you continue stirring frequently until you get the desired texture.

6. Transfer to a bowl and top it with fresh berries and coconut cream.

7. Serve warm or cold. Enjoy!

Keto Mushroom Omelet

Servings: 1

Ingredients:

- 3 mushrooms (washed and chopped)
- 3 eggs
- 1/5 yellow onion (chopped)
- 1 ounce shredded cheese
- 2 tablespoons butter
- Salt and pepper, to taste

Method:

1. Take a medium-sized bowl and crack the eggs into it. Add a pinch of pepper and salt to the cracked eggs.

2. Beat the eggs with a fork until they are frothy and smooth. Add more salt or pepper if required.

3. Melt the butter in a nonstick pan over medium heat.

4.   Pour the egg mixture into the melted butter and reduce the heat to low.

5.   Allow the omelet to cook for 3-4 minutes until the sides get firm.

6.   When the omelet still has a little rawness in the center, sprinkle the onions, cheese and mushrooms on the top.

7.   Carefully ease the edges of the omelet using a spatula and fold it over in half.

8.   Remove the pan from heat when the omelet turns golden brown and slide the cooked omelet onto a plate.

9.   Serve hot and enjoy!

Chapter Six: Vegetarian Keto Lunch Recipes

Crustless Spinach Cheese Pie

Servings: 8 slices

Ingredients:

- 10 ounces frozen (thawed, squeezed and drained) or fresh spinach (wilted down)

- 2 1/2 cups cheese (you can use any kind of full-fat cheese)

- 1/4 teaspoon garlic powder

- 5 eggs (beaten)

- 1 teaspoon minced onion (dried)

- Salt and pepper, to taste

- Nonstick cooking spray

Method:

1. Grease a 9-inch pie pan with nonstick cooking spray.

2. Preheat oven to 375 degrees Fahrenheit.

3. Take a medium-sized bowl and combine together the wilted down fresh spinach, cheese, garlic powder, beaten eggs, dried onion, salt and pepper.

4. Mix well until you get a batter-consistency mixture.

5. Pour this mixture into the greased pie pan and bake for 30 minutes until the edges brown.

6. Remove from the oven and let it cool. Slice the pie and transfer to a plate.

7. Serve warm and enjoy!

Rainbow Cauliflower Crust Pizza

Servings: 4

Ingredients:

- 3 cups cauliflower rice (1 small or medium-sized head of cauliflower should do)
- 1 cup diced bell peppers (combo of green, yellow, red, orange bell peppers)
- 1 egg
- 1/4 cup Parmesan cheese (shredded)
- 1/2 cup marinara sauce
- 1 1/4 cup mozzarella cheese
- 1/2 cup broccoli florets
- 1/2 teaspoon dry basil or minced rosemary
- 1/2 cup diced tomatoes
- 1/2 cup red onion (diced)
- 1/2 teaspoon dry oregano
- 1/4 teaspoon salt
- 1/2 teaspoon garlic powder

Method:

1. Preheat oven to 500 degrees Fahrenheit.

2. To make cauliflower rice, remove the cauliflower steps and cut the florets into chunks. Transfer the chunks to a food processor and pulse it until it looks like rice. You can also use a box grater or cheese grater.

3. Microwave the cauliflower rice on high for 5 minutes (use a microwave-safe bowl and don't cover the bowl). Remove the bowl and let it cool for 5 minutes.

4. Transfer the slightly cooled cauliflower onto a cheesecloth or kitchen towel. Squeeze out all the liquid carefully. Set aside.

5. Take a large bowl and crack the egg into it.

6. Add the cooked cauliflower, garlic powder, parmesan cheese, 1 cup mozzarella cheese, basil, oregano and salt into the bowl.

7. Mix thoroughly until all the ingredients are completely blended to form a dough mixture.

8. Line a parchment paper on a pizza pan and transfer the cauliflower mixture onto it.

9. Bake the cauliflower crust for 15 minutes until the crust turns crispy and golden brown.

10. Remove from the oven and top it with marinara sauce, remaining mozzarella cheese, broccoli florets, diced bell peppers and diced tomatoes.

11. Place the cauliflower crust pizza back into the oven and bake for another 15 minutes.

12. Once the pizza is ready, slice them and serve hot! Enjoy!

Roasted Brussels Sprouts with Pecans and Gorgonzola

Servings: 5

Ingredients:

- 1 1/2 pounds Brussels sprouts (fresh)
- 1/2 cup Gorgonzola cheese (crumbled) if you aren't using Gorgonzola, please use 2 tablespoons butter to toss the hot Brussels sprouts.
- 4 teaspoons + extra olive oil
- 1/2 cup chopped pecans
- Salt and black pepper (fresh ground), to taste

Method:

1. Preheat oven to 350 degrees Fahrenheit.
2. Grease the roasting pan with a small amount of olive oil using a paper towel or pastry brush. Set aside.

3. Trim the ends of Brussels sprouts and cut them lengthwise into halves. If they a bit large, cut them into fourths. If few leaves fall off, let it be.

4. Chop the pecans and set aside.

5. Take a small bowl and combine the chopped pecans and Brussels sprouts together.

6. Toss them with olive oil and season with fresh ground black pepper and salt. Be generous with your seasoning as there are no other spices.

7. Spread the coated pecans and Brussels sprouts on a roasting pan in a single layer.

8. Roast for 35 minutes until it browns and the sprouts turn tender. Keep stirring often to ensure they are evenly browned.

9. Remove from the oven and add the Gorgonzola cheese to the hot sprouts and pecans.

10. Toss them over before you serve and enjoy!

Charred Veggie and Fried Cheese Salad

Servings: 2

Ingredients:

- 1/2 cup sliced baby Portobello mushrooms
- 4 cups arugula, divided between 2 bowls
- 1 deseeded medium red bell pepper (cut into 8 pieces)
- 4 ounces goat cheese (cut into 4 ½ inch-thick medallions)
- 1 teaspoon garlic flakes
- 2 tablespoons poppy seeds
- 1 teaspoon onion flakes
- 2 tablespoons sesame seeds
- 1 tablespoon avocado oil
- Nonstick cooking spray

Method:

1. Take a small dish and combine together the garlic flakes, poppy seeds, onion flakes and sesame seeds.

2. Coat the goat cheese pieces with this flakes-seed mixture on both sides. Refrigerate until you are ready to fry them.

3. Grease a large skillet with nonstick cooking spray and heat to medium.

4. Char the mushrooms and pepper in the skillet until the pieces darken on both sides. The pepper should soften but charred well.

5. Take a large bowl and place the charred veggies in it. Add arugula to it and mix well.

6. Place the coated cheese in the same skillet and fry on both sides for 30 seconds as it melts quickly as you flip. So be gentle!

7. Add the fried cheese to the bowl and drizzle the avocado oil over it.

8. Serve the salad warm and enjoy!

Chapter Seven: Vegetarian Keto Dinner Recipes

5-Minute Keto Pizza

Servings: 1

Ingredients:

For the Pizza Crust

- 2 Eggs (large)
- 2 teaspoons olive oil
- 2 tablespoons Parmesan Cheese
- 1/2 teaspoon Italian Seasoning
- 1 tablespoon Psyllium Husk Powder
- Salt, to Taste

For the Toppings

- 1 tablespoon basil (freshly chopped)
- 1.5 ounces Mozzarella Cheese
- 3 tablespoons tomato Sauce

Method:

1. Take a medium-sized bowl and crack the eggs into it.

2. Add the Parmesan cheese, psyllium husk powder, olive oil, Italian seasoning and salt to the bowl.

3. Mix the ingredients using an immersion blender until all well-incorporated

4. Heat the olive oil in a large skillet over medium-high heat.

5. Pour a scoop of mixture into the hot skillet and spread it to a circle shape.

6. Cook for 60 seconds until the edges are brown. Flip and repeat. Remove from the stove.

7. Turn on the broiler and keep it ready.

8. Add the cheese and tomato sauce over the cooked pizza.

9. Broil for 2 minutes until the cheese bubbles.

10. Transfer to a plate and serve warm. Enjoy!

Cheese Cauliflower Casserole

Servings: 8

Ingredients:

- 1 cup shredded cheddar cheese,

- 1/2 medium onion (diced)

- 1 medium head cauliflower

- 1 cup sour cream

- Salt and pepper, to taste

- Nonstick cooking spray

Method:

1. Preheat the oven to 350 degrees Fahrenheit.

2. Grease the casserole dish with nonstick cooking spray and set aside.

3. Separate the stems and florets in the cauliflower. Chop them into small easy-to-bite pieces.

4. Transfer the chopped cauliflower to the greased cauliflower dish.

5.   Add the diced onions to the cauliflower and give it a toss.

6.   Pour the sour cream over the vegetables.

7.   Top it with cheese and mix the contents thoroughly until the well combined.

8.   Place the casserole dish in the oven and bake for 30 minutes.

9.   Transfer to a bowl and serve warm. Enjoy the creamy cheese cauliflower!

Vegetarian Lettuce Wraps

Servings: 4

Ingredients:

- 8 large butter lettuce leaves or inner romaine lettuce leaves from a romaine heart
- 8 ounces finely chopped cremini mushrooms
- 14 ounces extra-firm tofu (1 package) - do not use silken tofu
- 2 minced garlic cloves

- 8 ounces drained and finely chopped water chestnuts (1 can)
- 4 finely sliced green onions, divided
- 3 tablespoons soy sauce (reduced-sodium)
- 2 teaspoons ginger (freshly grated)
- 2 tablespoons rice vinegar
- 3 tablespoons hoisin sauce
- 1 teaspoon sesame oil
- 1/4 teaspoon red pepper flakes
- 2 teaspoons olive oil
- Grated carrots, for garnishing

Method:

1. Take a small bowl and mix together the sesame oil, hoisin sauce, rice vinegar and soy sauce thoroughly. Set it aside.

2. Squeeze out the liquid from the extra-firm tofu (you can press the tofu between paper towels and squeeze out the liquid).

3. Head the olive oil over medium-high heat in a large nonstick skillet.

4. Crumble the tofu on the hot oil and stir it well as it cooks. Break the large pieces into small ones. Allow it to cook for 5 minutes.

5. Add the mushrooms and stir the contents until the tofu blends well with the mushrooms.

6. Continue to cook for 4 minutes until the tofu turns golden brown and all the excess liquid from the tofu cooks off.

7. Add half of the green onions, ginger, garlic and water chestnuts to the skillet.

8. Cook for 30 seconds until the dish turns aromatic.

9. Pour the sauce mixture over and stir well until the contents are completely coated with the sauce.

10. Continue to cook for 1 minute until the liquid bubbles and sauce is completely heated through.

11. Place the lettuce leaves on a plate and place the cooked tofu-mushroom mixture on it.

12. Top it with grated carrots and remaining green onions. Repeat step 11 and 12 with the remaining lettuce leaves.

13. Serve immediately and enjoy!

Mediterranean Roasted Cabbage Steaks with Basil Pesto & Feta

Servings: 3-4

Ingredients:

- 1 small head cabbage (slice them into steaks)

- 2 ounces crumbled feta cheese,

- 4 ounces basil pesto

- 2 small tomatoes (sliced)

- 1 cup parmesan cheese (shredded)

- Fresh basil, for garnishing

- 1 tablespoon Mediterranean seasoning

- Olives, roasted red pepper (for topping)

- Nonstick cooking spray

Method:

1. Preheat oven to 400 degrees Fahrenheit.

2. Grease a large sheet pan with nonstick cooking spray (be generous while spraying the cooking spray).

3. Spread the cabbage steaks on the greased sheet pan and arrange them in a single layer.

4. Ensure the edges of the cabbage are touching each other.

5. Spread the basil pesto generously on the cabbage steak halves (you can slather more pesto as it will get into the folds of the cabbage when it melts).

6. Sprinkle the feta cheese on top followed by the sliced tomato and then the Parmesan cheese.

7. Bake them for 20 minutes until the cabbage edges turn crispy. You will also find the cheese all bubbling and melting.

8.   Remove from the oven and sprinkle the Mediterranean seasoning and fresh basil over it.

9.   Garnish with roasted red pepper and olives.

10.   Serve hot and enjoy!

Chapter Eight: Vegetarian Keto Snack Recipes

Crunchy Kale Chips

Servings: 2

Ingredients:

- 4 tablespoons olive oil

- 7 cups kale (loosely packed)

- 1/2 teaspoon salt

Method:

1. Preheat the oven to 325 degrees Fahrenheit.

2. Wash and rinse the kale thoroughly. Pat dry.

3. Remove the thick stems from the kale leaves and chop them.

4. Tear the leaves into large pieces.

5. Take a large bowl and place the chopped stems along with the torn kale leaves.

6.   Add 2 tablespoons of olive oil and mix well until the contents are completely coated with oil.

7.   Season it with salt and mix or toss it over.

8.   Grease a baking tray with 1 tablespoon olive oil and set aside.

9.   Spread the coated kale in the greased tray evenly. Ensure they are not crowded together.

10.   Bake for 10 to 15 minutes until the leaves and stems turn dry and crispy.

11.   Remove from oven and let it cool.

12.   Store in airtight containers and serve whenever needed.

Gluten-Free Crispy Buffalo Cauliflower Wings

Servings: 8

Ingredients:

For the Buffalo Cauliflower Wings

- 1/2 cup cassava flour

- 4 cups cauliflower florets

- 1 tablespoon hot sauce

- 2 teaspoons sea salt

- 1/2 cup filtered water

For the Buffalo Wing Sauce

- 2 minced garlic cloves

- 4 tablespoons hot sauce

- 2 tablespoons melted coconut oil

- 1 pinch sea salt, to taste

Method:

1. To make the buffalo wing sauce, take a small bowl and mix together the garlic, hot sauce, melted coconut oil and salt.

2. Stir well until the flavors are incorporated.

3. Heat a small skillet over medium-high heat. Pour the sauce mixture when the skillet is hot.

4. Reduce to medium-low heat and heat up the mixture for 5 minutes. Stir once in a while.

5. Remove from heat and set aside.

6. Preheat the oven to 450 degrees Fahrenheit.

7. Line a baking tray with parchment paper (unbleached).

8. If your cauliflower florets are large, cut them into bite-sized pieces.

9. Take another bowl and combine together the flour and salt.

10. Mix the hot sauce and filtered water well in another bowl.

11. Pour the sauce mixture into the flour and mix thoroughly. If the mixture is too thick, add a splash of water to make it into a thin consistency.

12. Coat each cauliflower florets with this sauce-flour batter and place them on the lined baking tray.

13. Ensure they are spread evenly and bake them for 30 minutes on the middle oven rack. Wait until they are crispy.

14. Drizzle with buffalo wing sauce and serve immediately. Enjoy!

Zucchini Nacho Chips

Servings: 4

Ingredients:

-   1 tablespoon healthy taco seasoning (low-carb)
-   1 large zucchini
-   4 tablespoons coconut oil

- Salt, to taste

Method:

1.   Slice the zucchini into thin strips using a mandoline slicer.

2.   Transfer these slices to a colander and place it onto a big plate.

3.   Sprinkle the zucchini slices with a lot of salt and let it sit for 5 minutes.

4.   Press out the water from the salted zucchini and set aside.

5.   Heat the oil over medium-high heat in a frying pan.

6.   Drop the zucchini in the hot oil and fry them.

7.   You should be able to fry 20 zucchini slices in one go.

8.   Remove from the pan once the zucchini turns crispy and golden brown.

9.   Place it on a plate lined with paper towels.

10.   Repeat steps 6 to 9 with the remaining zucchini slices.

11.   Sprinkle the taco seasoning over the fried zucchini and enjoy warm!

Cabbage Chips

Servings: 4

Ingredients:

- 1 cabbage head
- Sea salt, to taste

Method:

1.   Remove the core and separate the cabbage leaves.

2.   Wash and rinse thoroughly. Set it aside.

3.   Place the oven racks in the upper and lower thirds of the oven.

4.   Preheat the oven to 200 degrees Fahrenheit.

5. Boil water with salt in a large pot and cook the cabbage leaves in them for 2 minutes until it turns bright green and translucent.

6. Don't cook all the cabbage leaves in one go, you must work in batches by cooking 5 to 7 leaves every time.

7. Take a large bowl and fill it with ice water. Set aside.

8. Whenever the cabbage leaves are cooked, immediately transfer the cooked leaves using a large slotted spoon into the ice water bowl.

9. Let the leaves cool, drain them well and dry thoroughly.

10. Place a wire rack in rimmed baking sheets (the baking sheets should be large).

11. Now, arrange the cabbage leaves on the racks in one layer.

12. Bake for 3 hours until crisp and dry.

13. Toss it with salt and transfer to a bowl.

14. Serve warm and enjoy!

Crispy Green Bean Chips

Servings: 4

Ingredients:

- 5 pounds organic green beans (fresh or frozen)
- 1/4 cup nutritional yeast
- 1/3 cup melted coconut oil (or olive oil)
- 4 teaspoons salt

Method:

1. Blanch the beans if you are using fresh ones or thaw them if you are using frozen beans.

2. Take a large bowl and place the blanched or thawed green beans in it.

3. Preheat the oven to 250 degrees Fahrenheit.

4. Pour the coconut oil on top of the beans and mix them well with your hands.

5. Sprinkle the salt and nutritional yeast on top of the coated beans.

6.   Stir them well until the contents are well incorporated.

7.   Bake for 30 to 45 minutes until the beans become dry and crispy. (You can also bake in a low-temperature oven for 1 to 2 hours).

8.   Transfer to a plate and serve immediately.

Conclusion

We have come to the end of this book. I would like to take this opportunity to thank you once again for choosing this book.

The book discussed in brief about the ketogenic diet, vegetarian keto diet and the basic do's and don'ts in this dietary approach.

The chapters give brief detailing on the vegetarian ketogenic diet, health benefits of ketosis and the ways to get started with the keto-vegetarian diet. There are four chapters dedicated exclusively to delicious, healthy and tasty vegetarian keto recipes.

You can easily cook them and enjoy a sumptuous meal while your body takes up the responsibility of losing weight by turning into a fat-burning machine.

Eating tasty and healthy doesn't have to be boring anymore – it can be super fun!

Thank you and best wishes!